HAZARDS OF THE MOBILE PHONE &

WHAT YOU COULD DO TO PROTECT YOURSELF

MOBILE PHONE

SAFETY

....

MADHUKAR DAMA

Mobile Phone Safety
Hazards of the mobile phone &
What you could do to protect yourself

First Published 2014

This book contains information and advice on healthcare. It is
not intended, either in part or full, to replace medical advice. It
should not be used to replace the physician in case of health
issues. All the care has been taken to maintain the accuracy of
facts in this book, the publisher and author disclaim liability
for medical outcomes occurring as a result of application of the
suggested methods.

Contact: madhukar262@gmail.com

Cover Designed by Madhukar Dama using CreateSpace's
online cover designer
ISBN-13: 978-1495231223 (CreateSpace-Assigned)
ISBN-10: 1495231224

For Savitri and Adhya, the light of my eyes,
To Prof. H.A. Upendra, for guiding & supporting me,
&
To Rotary Kushalnagar, my real community

Contents

Author Preface

On the Christmas day of 2009, I was on cloud 9. Just a day before, I was engaged to Savitri and we were destined to marry in a couple of weeks. Next day, I travelled back to my laboratory at the Central Drug Research Institute, Lucknow. All these days, Savitri was not using a mobile phone. I insisted her to buy one so that we could talk and try to understand each other before marriage. We talked a few times daily, with last call of the lasting for more than half an hour every day.

On 9th of February 2010, we got married. This time I travelled back 1,000 miles to my laboratory with my wife. I resumed the work at the laboratory and working late was a routine for me. On such days, we had a few voice calls over mobile phones. After few months of this routine, Savitri started complaining about a strange sound she was hearing continuously. We checked with a doctor and she was diagnosed to be suffering from tinnitus, which receded after medication.

A week later, the strange sound returned and it was more painful this time. We checked again with a doctor and the sound disappeared after taking prescribed medication. However, the sound returned in some days.

This cycle continued for a few months. Meantime, a graduate student Neeraj Tiwari, who was conducting a large scale population survey on effects of mobile phone on subscribers at the Indian Toxicology Research Institute, approached me. Neeraj was interested to conduct a few studies in laboratory mice with my collaboration. He was basically an engineer and knew very less about laboratory mouse studies. As I was working on mice, he asked me to set up the experimental design. We designed and conducted studies on the effects of mobile phone on the reproductive system of male mice. During these days, he shared his findings about the myriad of effects of mobile phone use on the people of Lucknow city from his survey studies. Some experienced delusions, some had headaches, and some had difficulty in sleeping whereas some had ear problems.

I share many of the things I read or acquire with my wife. Most of the things Neeraj told me were passed on to Savitri. When I told her about the ear problems in mobile phone users, she intuitively decided that the sounds she was hearing were due to mobile phone use. We studied online about this and discussed it with Neeraj. We found that it was likely. Savitri stopped using a mobile phone to find out whether the sound will disappear. In a few days, it did. Ever since, she has stopped using a dedicated mobile phone and stays completely away from it.

With these events, I was motivated to conduct some studies on the effects of mobile phone. However, I neither had the equipments nor a laboratory. I pondered many months to find out ways to satisfy my needs to work on mobile phone hazards. A fine day, I thought of conducting an analysis of published papers to derive conclusions on the effects of mobile phone use on sperms. Such a study is called meta-analysis.

To my satisfaction, after analyzing all the suitable scientific studies published till 2012, I discovered that mobile phone use was significantly associated with deterioration in semen quality. Many important traits of the sperm quality like concentration, structure, motility, and viability were adversely deteriorated in mobile phone users. These effects were found when sperms were exposed to mobile phones in laboratory settings also.

I was thrilled to find proof for my ideas and published the findings in a peer reviewed research journal.

By this time, I was sure that mobile phones were hazardous and need to be used cautiously, better not to be used ever, especially by children and pregnant women. I came up with the idea of the 3 R's of mobile phone safety, which I shared with many. Most of the places I presented this idea, people shared their health issues which could be due to mobile phone use.

This motivated me to collect what I know and present in the form of a handy book that can be easily understood. So happened *Mobile Phone Safety*.

Madhukar Dama
26-March-2014

Chapter 1

The Largest Selling Hazard
in the History Of Mankind

*M*obile phone, also known as a cellular phone, mobile phone, or a hand phone, needs no introduction. Since its commercial availability in 1983, mobile phone has slowly but surely become a necessary gadget for all. The mobile phone was developed initially to make and receive telephone calls over a radio link while moving around a wide geographic area. Well, that is true no more as smartphones, which are an improved version of mobile phone, are hardly used for making calls anymore. From being a primary aim, making calls on mobile phones is now superseded by internet browsing, online socialization, listening to music, gaming, and texting.

In the 40 years since the first mobile phone call was made in 1973, the mobile phone has become the most ubiquitous consumer electronics device ever. During this time, the cost, capabilities, and size of mobile phones have changed dramatically to suit the needs and tastes of the consumers from all walks of life. In 1984, a mobile phone in the U.S. weighed over two pounds, cost nearly $4,000, and supported only one function: making calls. Today, an advanced phone with many enhancements is available for $20, whereas 8GB smartphones which are as smart as the curiosity rover are available for less than $200, weigh less than five ounces and can do things only dreamed of in 1984.

DynaTAC, the first cellular phone introduced by Motorola in 1983 was termed *portable radio telephone* by its manufacturer whereas people nicknamed it *The Brick*. The DynaTAC bears little resemblance to the mobile phones of today. *The Brick* was nine inches tall, weighed 790 grams, comprising 30 circuit boards and with a talk-time of 35 minutes. It took a whole 10 hours to recharge. Between then and now, handsets have undergone a dramatic evolution, changing as much in terms of design as they have on the features.

Major improvements in design, besides making them smaller, were the concept of flip-flop, touch screen, slide style, and wafer-thin large-screens, which transferred the car phones of the 1970s into the pocket phones of 1990s. Physical design innovations have led to advancements in camera quality, data download speed, and processing power more than anything else, which gave birth to the smartphones that have everything a person needs.

With the innovations in design, a lot of room was generated to expand the utility of a mobile phone. The earliest smartphone manufacturers experimented with providing users access to email, fax, pager, and address book. However, in recent years, the purpose of the mobile phone has shifted from a communication tool to a multimedia machine. We now buy a Smartphone not just to make calls, but to surf the web, check email, snap photos, and keep updated on social media. Innovations in design and features were complemented by the introduction of the app market that transformed the phone into a virtual toolbox with a solution for almost every need.

A basic Smartphone available in stores today can be used for making and receiving phone calls, texting, voicemail, accessing the Internet as well as a desktop computer, listening to music and watching videos, capturing pictures and videos. With the development of storage devices, memory of smartphones is now reaching enough to satisfy all the basic computing needs. Smartphone make use of small computer programs called apps that can perform a wide variety of functions for the user. Everything from looking up for weather conditions to finding the location of a nearest car garage is possible with these apps. Almost all smartphones are built with an ability to access a repository of thousands of apps making the functionality of smartphones almost limitless. Hence, a Smartphone can be considered as a communication device, a multimedia device, and a mini application operating platform rolled up all in a tiny pocket machine.

With all these innovations, a 150 gram smartphone has become twice as powerful as the 900 Kg Curiosity Rover, the most sophisticated spacecraft ever sent to another planet.

Innovations in mobile phones are having a great run at the cost of many other gadgets meant for core functioning, that have gradually become an integral part of the smartphone. The still camera and video recorder market is badly affected, as in addition to portability and the ability to shoot high quality pictures and videos, in a couple of clicks, and within a few seconds, media on the Smartphone can be shared with the world. Smartphones have also taken many other gadgets like personal video camera and players, portable music players, handheld gaming consoles, GPS devices, fixed line phones, pagers, wristwatches, alarm clocks, portable calculators, voice recorders, PDAs to the verge of extinction.

Seven Shades of Mobile, a study conducted by AOL and BBDO in 2012 over 30 days revealed the depth of integration of mobile phones in our life. Forty six percent of subscribers spend more than 850 minutes in a month on seeking relaxation or entertainment by watching a funny video, reading a gossip website, playing solitaire, or window-shopping on mobile. Nineteen percent subscribers used mobile for socializing (410 minutes a month), 12% used for shopping (126 minutes a month), 11% used for managing finance, health, and productivity (133 minutes a month), 7% used for planning (61 minutes a month), 4% used for seeking news and information (47 minute a month), and 1% used for participation in hobbies and interests (21 minutes a month). This study did not consider the time spent on voice calls, emails, and texting. Well, if we consider a subscriber who uses a mobile phone for all the 7 purposes, he will end up spending more than 27 hours in a month exclusively on his Smartphone. A recent analysis by Marcelo Ballve shows that the average U.S. smartphone owner spend about an hour of meaningful time on their device, while average U.S. app usage is two hours or more daily. This would roughly transform to 90 hours of time on a Smartphone every month. Is not that a significant amount of our life?

When these many conveniences are affordable, packed into a single device and can be carried effortlessly, it is hard not to imagine why a person cannot think of owning a mobile phone.

Nokia 1100, a far simple mobile phone according to today's standards, launched in 2003 shipped an incredible 250 million units and created a history by becoming the best selling consumer electronic device in the world. This feat has been repeated by numerous other mobile phone models since then.

As of now, there are more than 6.8 billion mobile subscriptions worldwide, estimates The International Telecommunication Union (February 2013). This figure represents a huge increase from 5.4 billion in 2010 through 6.0 billion in 2011, mostly due to the emergence of affordable smartphones. Putting the global population estimates at 7.1 billion, mobile phone subscriptions equal to 96 percent of the world population (7.1 billion according to the ITU).

Unlike global statistics, where mobile subscriptions are yet to increase, the developed world is witnessing saturation with subscriptions estimated at 128 per cent. On the contrary, mobile phone penetration in developing nations and Africa is around 89 percent and 63 percent of the population respectively, according to the ITU. The subscriptions seem to be neither stabilized nor declining as mobile Factbook 2013 (Portio Research) has predicted that mobile subscriptions will reach 7.5 billion by the end of 2014 and 8.5 billion by the end of 2016. Due to large population base, over half of the mobile subscribers are in Asia Pacific. Africa and Middle East have also adopted the mobile phones for daily use, which will eventually lead to increases in subscription base by 2016 to reach the second highest in number.

Mobile subscriptions refer to the number of SIM cards being used in each country, not the number of people using a mobile device. Some people have two mobile accounts on the go at a time, which could be carried by two different mobile phone sets or in a single dual-SIM device. Wireless Intelligence (October 2012) estimates that consumers use on average 1.85 SIM cards each, which brings down the number of unique mobile users worldwide at any given time by 45 percent.

With this much of dependence on and ability to perform an unlimited number of activities, mobile phone is ranked 1st on the list of all time gadgets and is considered the most important gadget in history of mankind.

Wait; there is a cache!

Mobile phones are indispensable, but are they safe?

Not likely, as the following points make it clear.

- On 31 May 2011 the International Agency for Research on Cancer (IARC) classified radiofrequency electromagnetic fields, on which mobile phones operate, as possibly carcinogenic to humans (Group 2B). This means that mobile phones carry similar risk as exposure to lead, the pesticide DDT and petrol exhausts.

- Mobile phone manuals advise subscribers to keep the device away from the body, even when the device is not in use.
- Mobile phone users are likely to become infertile.
- Mobile phone use is now implicated in at least 25% of all car crashes.
- Mobile phones are banned from school premises as they could affect learning as well as health of children.

These are some of the health hazards which a mobile user could get affected by. The mobile phone stays connected with its mast through microwave radiation at levels that could, over a period of time, get absorbed into the body, disrupt the DNA, weaken the brain's protective barrier and release highly reactive and damaging free radicals. That is how mobile phones can damage our cells.

Everybody seems to own a mobile phone; that does not mean they are innocuous. History is staring at us with examples of things we used routinely, from tobacco to trans-fats to mercury, only to learn eventually of the precarious lunacy in which we were engaged.

Well, enough evidence has accumulated and it is time to convince ourselves that the largest selling gadget in the history of humanity is not as safe as we have believed!

ⅪⅪⅪⅪⅪ

The Ever Exploding Hazard

*C*ell phones got their name from the way the system of wireless communication works. The cell is the major component of the mobile phone system. The area of service covered for communication is divided into a set of cells that looks like a hexagonal grid, with the base station or phone tower installed at its center. The tower typically covers an area of 2 to 3 square miles in all the directions. A handheld cellular phone is communicated by the base tower once every ten minutes, even when calls are not made. When the subscriber moves away from the coverage area of a base tower, the subscriber is transferred over to the next base tower. An area of operation has hundreds of towers which are connected to the mobile telephone switching office (MTSO) where mobile calls are routed to the receivers. When a subscriber places call while moving, the system hands off the connection to the next cell tower, keeping the connection live which provides for uninterrupted voice calls and data transfer on the go.

When a mobile phone is turned on, it identifies the programmed frequencies and connects with the nearest base station; or else, if it is out of range it will display a 'no service' message. If connection succeeds, the MTSO registers it and start tracking subscriber's location within the cell. On placing a call, the MTSO receives the call and switches it to the service provider of the receiver. After this the call can theoretically go on forever. As the subscriber move towards the edge of the cell, the MTSO notes the diminishing strength of signal and immediately hand over the subscriber to the next cell.

Anatomically, mobile phone is a very simple device. The mobile phone contains just a few individual parts, a display, an antenna, a microphone, a keyboard, a battery, a speaker, and a circuit board with the microprocessor which is the heart of the system. The microprocessor handles all the functions from integrating with keyboard and display to communicating with the base tower to coordinate the rest of the functions. The memory devices provide storage for the operating system, contacts and media files, whereas radio and power section deals with power management and recharging. The radio frequency amplifiers channel the signal coming in and going out of the device. This tiny setup ensures conversion of the sound waves into digital codes that are transmitted to the MTSO which in turn delivers it to the receiver via his service provider without loss of fidelity.

The digital signal transmitted between the mobile phone and the base station is based on microwave radiation (radiofrequency radiation). The base stations are a matter of public health concern. However, base towers may not be as harmful as handheld mobile devices if they are located at a proper distance.

On contact with a material, microwave radiations transmit their energy and become weaker. The absorption depends on the frequency, property and the size of the contact material. This is the reason, the scientists fear for the ability of mobile phones to cause brain tumors, especially in children. Three fourth of the human brain is formed by water and skull of children are not as thick as adults. As microwaves have a high affinity for water molecules, scientists fear of mobile phone users getting brain cancers is justified.

The safety of the mobile phones, expressed as the Specific Absorption Rate (SAR), is currently determined by the rate at which energy is absorbed by the human body when exposed to its radio frequency (RF) electromagnetic field. The International Commission on Non-Ionizing Radiation Protection (ICNIRP) has recommended limits for SAR, based on the knowledge that an exposure of the whole body with an average SAR of 4 W/kg will lead to a temperature rise of 1 °C. Whole body exposure limits are set ten to fifty times below this level with a rationale that no heating will occur in the human body. These criteria have been found to work well and heating if any, in the brain of the mobile phone user was found to remain below 0.1 °C. A small rise of temperature is considered physiologically harmless.

Unfortunately, there is a potential for long-term cumulative microwave absorption that could produce non-thermal effects.

Mobile phones with a potential to heat human tissues up to 1 °C are considered safe;

however, there are numerous studies which have established that even at this level of heating, some of the tissue like eyes and testes could be irreversibly damaged.

Most of the mobile phones in the market and base towers adhere to the safety guidelines. There is no question of hazards due to thermal effects of mobile radiation. However, thousands of research studies have documented adverse health effects in mobile phone users, which is possibly due to non-thermal effects which we cannot measure on a temperature scale.

Hundreds of incidences of hazards in mobile phone users like radiation hypersensitivity, genetic damage, reproductive problems, behavioral and developmental problems in children, brain dysfunction and tumors of various organs are revealed by scientific studies. This is a window to the grave problems that we are about to welcome if this issue is not addressed. It is hardly a decade that mobile phones have entered the hands of many and we have so many instances of the health problems. The situation is not going to improve if the exposure to microwave radiation continue this way, and it will not be uncommon to witness a global epidemic of a myriad of health problems in near future.

The human body has evolved numerous ways to identify the radiations and waves and has its own methods to respond. Our organs, especially the heart and brain use electrical signals to convey information. Some of the electrical activities operate with frequency that are similar to the microwaves emitted from mobile phone signals. Thus, our body may respond to the absorbed microwaves considering it to be a normal internal signal. This could give rise to a variety of non-thermal effect based on the body area involved. One elegant example that could be dug from the archives of medical paradoxes is flashing of a light at a frequency similar to that of the brain can produce a type of seizure called photosensitive epilepsy. Interestingly, the energy of the light bulb is no concern here; rather it is the regularity of flashing that deceives brain to perceive it as a signal to go epileptic.

A 2013 survey by mobile phone provider O2 showed that in a day, an average user, spend 24 minutes browsing the internet, 16 minutes checking social networks, 15 minutes listening to music, 13 minutes each playing games and making calls, 11 minutes texting, 9 minutes on emails, 8 minutes reading books, 7 minutes watching TV/films, and 3 minutes taking photographs. In addition to this, the phone is carried on the body all the time and put nearby while sleeping

This means that we are continually bombarded with the harmful microwaves from our favorite gadget!

ⵣⵣⵣⵣ

Chapter 3

Myriad of Effects

 he World Health Organization (WHO) defined health in its broader sense in 1946 as "a state of complete physical, mental, and social well-being and not merely the absence of disease or infirmity. Mobile phones happen to affect humans physically, mentally and socially in numerous ways. I would like to throw light on some of the most common effects of mobile phone that have been proven by scientific studies.

Fitness

Fitness is a layman's synonym for health. A person can be called 'fit' if he is not carrying any physical injury/deformity, mental problems and behaves in a socially acceptable way. Fitness reflects nutritional status, physical condition, hygiene practices, and rest by the body. All healthy persons can be considered fit and vice versa. However, health and sports writers use the term 'fitness' as a synonym for the physical attributes of the individual. An individual can maintain his fitness through regular exercise, balanced diet, hygiene, moral behavior, and by providing proper rest to the body.

Today's phones, especially the smartphones provide unlimited access to information and activities through apps and on the go access to the internet. This keeps the user hooked to his phone. The time spent on screen equals to lack of physical activity. Studies on college students have supported the negative relation of phone use and overall fitness, most likely due to increased sedentary position as well as exposure to microwave radiations.

Joint problems

We have joints all over the body that helps us make movements. Each bone is connected with its adjacent bone through a joint. Hence, a joint is the interface of the surface of two bones, a cavity that separates the bones, and the joint capsule that holds the ends together. The cavity is sealed from all the side by joint capsule. The cavity contains a lubricating fluid called synovial fluid that reduces the friction on all the structures in the joint.

When the joints are used regularly, the lubrication is maintained, the fibrous materials remain active and strong due to reflex action. If a joint is not moved for a longer period of time, the fibers get shortened, the capsule shrinks and the mobility of the joint is reduced. This is the reason for advocating physiotherapy and exercise to maintain joint health. Flexibility of the joint depends on age and health status of a person. As a rule, joint flexibility varies from person to person. The best way to maintain the health of joint is by intake of balanced diet and regular stretching exercise. Proper rest is also as important as exercise.

Imagine standing with the empty palm held to ear for fifteen minutes. It is very difficult to do so. One thing is it is boring and second the elbow starts paining after few minutes. Texting, calling and playing games on mobile phones put the elbows and finger joints to work. As we are hooked on to the call or the information, we tend to neglect the pain in the elbow. But the joint is physically immobilized for the duration of the mobile phone use. Holding phone to the ear also puts strain on the neck. The elbow aches experienced by mobile phone users are referred as "mobile phone elbow."

Not every mobile phone user may get the 'mobile phone elbow' same way. Some are more prone than others due to duration of use and style of holding the phone. The pain may not be continuous. It starts initially after holding the phone for calls and then the pain could remain even after a long time. If untreated, it may lead to loss of fine motor skills and in extreme situation may end up with paralysis. Holding a phone to the ear with the elbow flexed can aggravate other elbow related problems like Cubital Tunnel Syndrome.

Fingers of texting users are affected due to a different reason altogether. Our motor muscles have an extent of contraction and relaxation. After a full contraction, a full relaxation should follow to relax the muscle and help it recover. Texting on mobile phone requires repeated small muscle movements that do not stretch the muscle over its entire range. This does not give the muscle a chance to relax. This leads to stiff fingers. If unattended, this could also lead to numbness and irreversible damage in the finger joints.

Hearing loss

Unlike nose, tongue and eyes, which use chemical method of communication, ears use a completely mechanical process to pick up the sound and translate it into a form that the brain can infer. All the parts of the ear play important and distinct roles in hearing. The outer ear composed of the external ear and the ear canal collects the noise from the surroundings, the middle ear formed by the ear drum and three very small bones transmits the sound waves captured by external ear to the inner ear with maximum fidelity, and the inner ear composed of the sensory tiny hairs and auditory nerve converts the sound vibrations and conveys it to the brain by electrical impulses.

Hearing can be impaired if the sensory cells and fibers are exposed frequently to louder sounds. A very loud sound can cause hearing loss on a short exposure by irreversibly damaging the sensory cells and fibers. Whereas frequent vibrations due to continuous exposure to noise can gradually lead to hearing loss due to inability of damaged cells to rest and heal. Loss of the vision and hearing loss are different. Deterioration of vision makes reading harder as the letters get smaller, but hearing loss can make certain high pitched syllables and sounds uninterpretable.

Noise pollution is the most common occupational hazard we are facing today. More than 360 million people in the world are living with one or the other type of hearing loss. A common and usually first bad experience of mobile phone users is a warm feeling, ringing or a clogged feeling in the ear after a long voice call. Studies have shown that using a mobile phone for more than an hour a day could damage hearing. Young adult mobile phone users have been found to face difficulty in hearing words starting with the letters s, f, h, t and z. The problem was particularly noticeable in the right ear, after a regular use of the mobile phone over a period of four years. Inability to distinguish high-frequency syllables like s, f, h, t and z, can make it difficult to differentiate common words like hill, fill and till.

Ringing ear (Tinnitus)

Tinnitus is a common ear problem with limited treatment options, wherein one feels a ringing or booming sensation in one or both ears. A study published in a British journal reported that the chances of a subscriber getting tinnitus doubles after four years of mobile phone use. Further, this study also showed that a person using mobile phone before onset of tinnitus is 37% more likely to get the condition and mobile phone use for as low as 10 minutes a day increases the likelihood of tinnitus by 71%. The absorption of microwave radiations by the ear has been suggested as a possible basis of this association. However, it is also likely that holding a mobile phone close to ear during voice calls over a period of time, thereby continuously bombarding the inner ear with sound waves, could cause this problem.

Eye damage

The human eye is a self adjusting camera. Cornea, the transparent portion in the very front of the eye focuses the light falling on the eye. Iris, a colored ring shaped membrane behind the cornea controls the amount of light entering into eyes through an adjustable opening called pupil. Just behind the pupil the transparent lens is located. The space formed between the cornea and the iris is filled by a clear fluid called the aqueous humor. Inside of the eye is filled with a jelly-like substance called vitreous humor. Light entering through cornea, passes through pupil and the lens and falls on the highly sensitive layer of cells called the retina. The retina sends the information received through the light to the brain which ultimately visualizes the colors and shapes seen.

When a mobile phone is used, especially for a longer duration for playing games and watching videos or reading, the light as well as microwave radiations enter into the eyes and generate a small amount of heat, similar to the way a microwave oven cooks the meat. Unlike heating in other parts of the body, the excess heat cannot be easily removed from the eyes, as eyes have fewer blood vessels than other organs, which renders it difficult to lose heat. Continuous staring at mobile phones reduces the number of eye blinks which can dry the eyes leading to irritation, burning sensation and damage.

Laboratory tests have showed that the eye lens of calves looses the ability to focus clearly on a beam of light and develop bubbles on exposure to mobile phone radiation, which indicates a permanent damage that could ultimately lead to cataract.

Headache and migraine

Mobile phone user's frequently get headache, especially after prolonged voice calls. Several scientific studies have examined this relation and showed that users who read extensively on Smartphone are likely to get migraine, headache and eyestrain.

Constantly looking at mobile phone screen during texting, gaming, and reading force our eye to focus rapidly, for which eyes are not accustomed. This leads to problems with vergence, the ability of eyes to focus from near to far objects. Prolonged use of mobile phone reduces the eye's ability to vergence; triggering headache, migraine or nausea. The headache may not be caused solely due to radiation. The ergonomics of mobile phone handling or the heat from the phone could also trigger it. Other studies have suggested that sleep loss due to mobile phone use could also trigger headache due to fatigue and tiredness.

Pedestrian injury

More than 1,500 pedestrians were admitted to emergency treatment hospital wards in 2010 for injuries arising out of distracted walking due to use of a mobile phone in the United States. This figure may be a significant underestimate as mobile phone users often do not attribute the injuries to distraction and may not approach emergency wards for treatments. Injuries to the mobile phone using pedestrian are estimated to double by 2015. Strange varieties of injuries were reported ranging from a fall into 8 feet deep ditch leading to chest and shoulder injuries to getting knocked down by a car. The authors of the study estimated that more than 2 million individuals may be injured by mobile phone related distraction while commuting.

Fatigue

Fatigue, characterized by a temporary state of tiredness, listlessness, and laziness occurs as a result of mental or physical exhaustion, usually at the end of a long day. Fatigue can be caused by many factors. Fatigue is a symptom as it is a subjective feeling which is experienced in self but may not be easily appreciated in others. Fatigue can be overcome by rest. However, improper or insufficient rest or sleep can lead to fatigue.

Sleep deprivation kills a human faster than food deprivation, as a daily dose of 6-8 hours of sound sleep is absolutely necessary for restoration of the body from everyday wear and tear. A proper sleep-wake cycle is maintained by the duration and amount of light entering into the eyes. Melatonin, a hormone that regulates sleep is highly responsive to light. The light from sun keeps us awake and sunset makes us sleep naturally.

A study conducted by Sara Thomee and her colleagues on over 4000 adults aged between 20 to 24 years showed that intensive use of mobile phones can lead to sleep disorders. Further, men were specifically more prone to sleep disorders. With the use of gadgets like television, computer and mobile phones, especially during night times, our eyes are exposed to light well beyond the normal durations we are adapted to. This disrupts melatonin production, throws off circadian rhythm, and prevents sleep and lead to fatigue the next day. It is not only the exposure to light, but physical strain due to staying in an uncomfortable posture during mobile phone use, especially while playing games and making long calls, that combines with melatonin disruption leading to fatigue.

Skin allergy

Metals used in the mobile phone can initiate skin allergies!

Nickel is used extensively in mobile phones for handset, screen and buttons. Studies have shown that about one third of humans are likely to be sensitive to nickel. These people could develop skin allergies on contact with the mobile phone leading to inflammation, blisters, dryness and cracks. Nickel coated jewelry are a common cause of dermatitis in women. When such women are exposed to nickel in mobile phones, dermatitis could flare up. This makes women particularly more susceptible to nickel allergies.

Nearly half of all the mobile phones in the market and most of the fashionable models carry free nickel on the menu buttons, logos, and frame of the display screen. A typical allergic reaction can happen on skin and area around the ear and neck.

If you get an allergic rash on face or hands, it's time to consider the mobile phone as a very likely cause.

Weakening of the Blood brain barrier & changes in the brain activity

Between the actual brain tissue and the blood that circulates in the brain is a fine cell layer called blood brain barrier (BBB), that selectively permits nutrients while prevents entry of numerous poisonous and harmful substances into the brain cells. The BBB is absolutely necessary to protect our brain from numerous harmful chemicals circulating in the blood.

Damage to the BBB is like bringing the brain outside the body as it will be freely exposed to unwanted chemicals. Many lethal and debilitating diseases are produced when BBB is damaged like meningitis, brain abscess, epilepsy, multiple sclerosis, sleeping sickness, Alzheimer's disease and cerebral edema.

Cellular phone increases the porosity of the BBB!

Studies conducted in laboratory rats have shown that albumin proteins, which are filtered by the BBB, can penetrate into brain after exposure to mobile phones. The amount of albumin entering the brain was small but sufficient enough to kill the brain cells.

Similar exposure of the cells from the human brain blood vessels to microwaves at the maximum legal limit has revealed an alteration of thousands of chemicals. American soldiers involved in Kuwait war have suffered unexplained symptoms, which are now believed to be due to heavy use of microwave based high tech instruments that could have damaged the BBB leading to absorption of toxin by brain cells.

A recent study published in the prestigious journal JAMA based on work conducted at the National Institute of Health reported that less than an hour of mobile phone use can speed up brain activity in the area nearest to the phone antenna. This was the first and largest study to document that the brain activity could be altered even after a short duration exposure to the mobile phone.

Erectile dysfunction

Humans are sexually reproducing species and penis is indispensible for procreation. But copulation cannot be done without erection of the penis. Erection of the penis is a complex phenomenon and requires the man to be in good health. An erection begins in the brain. On visual, physical or mental stimulation for intercourse, brain sends chemical signals to the penis. Upon receiving these signals, the chambers in penis starts trapping blood and gets engorged, leading to erection which can be sustained until stimuli persists or ejaculation is achieved.

As erection require a complex sequence of events, many factors can lead to erectile dysfunction (ED) which is essentially a failure of the penis to trap the blood. Some of the common causes of ED are anti-depressants, nicotine, neurogenic disorders, penile disorders, psychological causes like performance anxiety, stress, mental disorders, negative feelings, surgery, ageing, kidney failure, chronic diseases such as diabetes and multiple sclerosis, and lifestyle factors like smoking and obesity.

In an article from the 2012 Proceeding of the

World Meeting on Sexual Medicine, men having difficulty with erection were found to be 2.6 times more likely to carry mobile phone in their trousers.

Male infertility

Sperm has evolved to play a single yet indispensable role, that is to deliver the genetic materials of man to the egg with utmost fidelity. This is achieved with the help of the testes and the seminal fluid both of which maintains the quantity, quality and motility of sperms necessary to achieve fertilization. Hence any effects on these parameters will prevent a man from reproducing.

More than 15% of the human couples are infertile! The incidence is increasing day by day.

Experiments on the effects of mobile phone radiations have been conducted since at least 2003. From these studies on rats to very recent studies conducted on humans, a very strong connection has been scientifically established between the mobile phones and male infertility. In fact, Ashok Agarwal, who is a leading researcher on human sperms, calls the mobile phones as "nemesis of the modern man". Men using mobile phones have been found to produce lower number of sperms, with poor structural and motility capacity, carrying a damaged genetic material.

Sleep disturbance, confusion, mood swings, stress & depression

Sleep is a multistage activity with different but essential repairs occurring at these stages. The first stage called non-rapid eye movement (REM) stage consists of the interim period between wakefulness and sleep (sub-phase 1) up to initiation of the actual sleep (sub-phase 2). The second stage, known as deep-REM phase consists solely of sleep wherein repair of the bone and skin (sub phase 1) occurs in addition to restoration of physical energy by increased flow of blood to the musculature (sub phase 2). Third stage called REM sleep starts only after 90 minutes of continuous sleep and is characterized by very deep sleep and vivid dreams.

A 2008 report published at the MITs Progress in Electromagnetics Research Symposium which was funded by the Mobile Manufacturers Forum, provided comprehensive evidence that mobile phones, especially when used during late nights, affects sleep pattern, and causes headaches and confusion. The deeper stages of sleep, which is most essential was both delayed as well as reduced. This interferes with the body's ability to repair daytime exhaustions and could lead to personality changes, ADHD like symptoms in children, lack of concentration, depression, mood swings and poor academic performance. More than three quarters of young people keep their mobile phones at the hands reach, or below the pillow during sleep. And mobile phone has become the new alarm clock!

Annoyance and distraction

Mobile phone in everybody's hand with a high probability of getting a call anytime means that we are exposing our as well as everybody else's privacy and peace of mind. When a mobile phone rings in a public place, a few people at least instantly take a look at their phone only to realize that it is not their phone that is ringing. This phenomenon has become popular as ringxiety. Further, we encounter at least a few subscribers daily who make sure that everybody on the street or the hall knows every word they speak on the mobile phone.

Is that not very annoying!

A study has proved that overhearing a mobile phone conversation is much more demanding than listening to a face to face conversation!

Distracted driving and traffic accidents

Driving requires 100% focus, else death is possible!

Driving is distracted by taking off the hands from the wheel, taking off the eyes from the road and taking off the brain from the driving. Using a mobile phone during driving can lead to all the three types of distractions. Distraction is mainly caused by acts of looking after children, texting, talking on the phone or to a passenger, eating, or reading while driving. Distracted driving endangers the safety of the driver, passengers, bystanders and those in other vehicles.

A visit to Edgar Snyder and Associates websites reveals very interesting statistics on mobile phone use during driving like

- *The chances of a crash are increased by 4 times by talking on mobile phone and 23 times by texting.*

- *The reaction time of a young driver talking on a mobile phone is lowered to an extent that it is comparable to that of a 70 year old man.*

- *Texting while driving takes the attention away for a period of time by which the vehicle would have traversed a distance of a football field.*

- *94% of drivers support bans on texting while driving, whereas 74% of drivers support bans on hand-held mobile phone use.*

- *In 2012, about 421,000 people were injured in crashes involving a distracted driver in United States.*

- *The Transportation Safety Group found that distracted drivers account for nearly 80 percent of car crashes.*

Despite these apparent dangers and willingness to support the ban on distracted driving, more than 80% of the drivers either use a mobile phone or indulge in texting while driving!

More than 100 nations have banned the use of mobile phone while driving.

Killing communication skills

Nearly, one in ten children get their first mobile phone at age 5 and an average age for owning a first mobile phone is around 11 years!

The young children are getting more versed in using texting lingo before they could learn proper English and one-on-one conversation skills. This will eventually affect the acquisition of proper language skills need to be learnt at later ages.

Texting removes the need for face to face or voice communication which requires more efforts as there is need for understanding the depth of the words by interpreting body language, expression and characters of the voice. But this is absolutely necessary to learn the concept of communication as more than 80% of the communications happen through body language.

Each human has a unique personality which is defined by his body language! Texting has no personality. Except the message, it carries nothing for the benefit of receiver.

The more we text for communication, the less we will be able to interpret subtle aspects of communication. I am worried; my children may not be able to make meaningful eye contacts if they become the slaves of texting at an early age.

Affecting socialization

Socialization is a lifelong process of acquiring and spreading habits, norms, customs, ideologies, and skills that are necessary for an individual to participate meaningfully in his own society. Socialization is necessary, en mass, for maintaining moral values in a society.

Effective socialization requires face to face communication.

However, a study by Pew Research Centre showed that almost 13 % of the Americans pretend to be using a mobile phone to avoid interaction with someone.

A study by Scott Campbell, published in the journal *Human Communication Research*, studied more than 1800 subscribers and found that frequency and style of mobile phone use is affecting the way we are interacting with others.

People who talk on mobile phones frequently are less likely to communicate in public.

Though mobile phones have increased regular contacts with near ones, they are reducing the face to face contacts with strangers, which will reduce the ability of our next generation to read faces and understand subtle meanings conveyed by body language.

Predisposition to Selfishness & Criminality

A study by Anastasiya Pocheptsova and her colleagues at the University of Maryland found that a short period of mobile phone use decreased willingness of the teenagers to volunteer for a community service activity. Interestingly, this antisocial behaviour was even triggered by just sketching a picture of their mobile phone. The authors attributed this behaviour to ability of the mobile phone to evoke feelings of connectivity to others, which fulfils the basic desire to *belong*.

In a three year study conducted on 2,300 students at the University of Winnipeg, very interesting results were discovered about the relation of texting habits and behaviour of the teenagers. Teenagers who texted more than 100 times a day tended to place less importance on moral, aesthetic and spiritual goals, and greater importance on wealth and image. Further, the most incessant texters were also likely to be slightly more racist than others. About 2% of the text messages were antisocial which were found to be sent by antisocial teenagers.

Behavioural problems

About 18 % of the children are exposed to mobile phones before and after birth, and 35 % of 7 year olds use a mobile phone.

Researchers from the School of Public Health at the University of California, Los Angeles studied more than 28,000 children and found that, by the age of 7, children exposed to mobile phones before and after birth were two times more likely to suffer from emotional or behavioural problems as compared to the children who were not exposed to the phones. Further, children not exposed to mobile phones during this time, but using it by 7 years of age had a 20% more likelihood of behavioural problems.

A earlier study by these authors had revealed that children using mobile phone are 80 percent more likely to suffer from difficulties with behaviour, 25 percent more at risk from emotional problems, 34 percent more likely to suffer from difficulties relating to their peers, 35 percent more likely to be hyperactive and 49 percent more prone to problems with conduct.

I would like to stress on the fact that fetal/children skull is much more thinner compared to adult and a similar duration of exposure to mobile phone microwaves is much more dangerous to children. Experiments have shown that the brains of young ones absorb more than double amount of microwaves compared to an adult brain.

Cancers

A large number of studies suggest a link between mobile phone towers or mobile phones and a variety of cancer. However, an equal number of studies contradict this.

A large body of evidence for the ability of mobile phone radiations to induce cancer is published, but is still equivocal!

The World Health Organization is still weighing the evidence in support of the carcinogenic potential of mobile phones, which is a major concern of subscribers as well as many scientists. However, it must be noted that, in the year 2012, the International Agency for Research on Cancer (a constituent body of WHO) has declared mobile phones as possibly carcinogenic (Group 2B) based on available literature.

¤¤¤¤¤

Chapter 4

3 R's of Safety

Do Cellphones Cause Brain Cancer? Read a headline of a New York Times website on April 13, 2011

Cellphone Radiation May Cause Cancer, Advisory Panel Says, was the headline of a New York Times story on May 31, 2011

No Cellphone-Cancer Link in Large Study, was titled a story in the New York Times on October 20, 2011

In a year, between few months a reader is bombarded with totally contradictory research findings about the possibility of mobile phone use leading to the development of cancer. I expect this confusion to run for many more years to come as cancer is a very atypical disorder and mobile phones have arrived very recently.

If we assume that mobile phones cause cancer, we need to take precautions!

If we assume that mobile phones are likely to cause cancer, we need to take precautions!

However, if we assume that mobile phones are not likely to cause cancer, we still need to take precautions. This is because the myriads of effects presented in the previous section have been supported unequivocally by scientific studies.

Whether mobile phone use lead to cancer remains to be agreed upon, but nobody can argue that they are safe.

Internet search on mobile phone safety retrieves numerous WebPages providing a variety of advise. A visit to these WebPages reveals that the advices are either incomplete, unscientific or are intended to sell a so called safety product which may further damage the health of subscribers. Hence, I have developed a concept of "Rule of 3 R's" for the safety of mobile phone users. The 3 R's are a compilation of the scientifically sound preventive measures to minimize the hazards to the mobile phone user to the lowest possible extent.

Rule 1 – **R**eplacement

Most of the time mobile phones are used not because it is necessary, but because it is available. It is possible to overcome this habit by switching to other means of communication to prevent exposure to the microwave radiations. Land phones which use wired connections and voice over internet protocol programs (VoIP) like Skype, Gtalk etc. are good alternatives to mobile phones. Similarly, desktop computers can be used to access internet services instead of mobile phones. These measures can reduce exposure to mobile phones at home or workplace. Switching to safer alternatives is the best method; however mobile phone use is unavoidable outdoors, where the user can reduce exposure by reducing and refining the usage.

Rule 2 – **R**eduction

Mobile phone users can reduce the exposure to radiations drastically by using a branded product with minimal value of specific absorption rate (SAR). Further reduction can be achieved by switching off during sleep and long periods of unuse, by not wearing the phone on the body, by making small calls, and by texting instead of a voice call.

Rule 3 – Refinement

A manner in which mobile phone is used also dictates the amount of radiation absorbed by the body. Poor quality signal or weak battery increases the exposure drastically as mobile phone has to work hard to maintain the quality of the call. Mobile phone use should be avoided when battery is low or signal is weak. To prevent damage to the ears as well as reduce absorption of radiation into the brain, mobile phone should not be kept pressed to ears and speaker function or wired earphone should be used. To protect eyes, staring for long hours at the mobile phone screen should be avoided. Mobile phone use should be avoided around other electronic appliances or metal fittings as it increases or focuses the radiations. Open and empty spaces should be preferred to make longer calls. The metal components of spectacle frames, zipper, undergarments which are worn on the body can focus signals which can increase the exposure of specific organ to a higher level. Similarly a person with medical fittings like a pacemaker, tooth filling, or knee implant should be careful not to allow mobile phone interferes with the implants. Owning multiple mobiles or using multiple SIM card fitted phones drastically increases exposure to radiations. A mobile phone with single SIM card and user safety features should be preferred. The mobile phone should not be used inside a moving vehicle as the mobile phone signal intensity changes with distance from base tower and the metal body of the vehicle traps the signal, which ultimately increases the exposure levels. Using mobile phone reduces the concentration on other activities, which is proven by numerous studies to be a major risk factor for traffic accidents. The National Safety Council estimates that at least 1.6 million crashes are caused each year by drivers using mobile phones and texting.

Though I am sure that the 3 R's can reduce the health hazards by limiting cumulative absorption of microwave radiation in adult subscribers, it is necessary to completely refrain from mobile phone use for children as their brains absorb relatively higher amount of radiations which coupled with the possibility of long term lifetime exposure may lead to serious health effects with age. Similarly, pregnant women should refrain from mobile use as it is shown to produce a variety of defects in the children.

¤¤¤¤¤

Chapter 5

Take Home Message

1. Mobile phones are not safe!
2. World Health Organization has classified electromagnetic radiations emitted by mobile phones as *possibly carcinogenic.*
3. Replace the mobile phone with safer alternatives like wired landphone or voice over internet protocol programmes (VoiP) like Skype, Gtalk etc, whenever possible.
4. Use desktop computer to access internet services.
5. Use a good quality mobile phone with smaller values of specific absorption rate (SAR). Mobile phones have SAR values ranging from a low of 0.1 to a high of 1.9. Using phones with lower SAR will drastically reduce the exposure to radiations.

6. Switch off the mobile phone during sleep and long periods of unused.

7. Do not carry mobile phone in pockets or bras. Keep the phone away from the body.

8. Make smaller calls.

9. Prefer texting over voice call.

10. Do not use mobile phone when signal is weak.

11. Do not use mobile phone when battery is low. Keep battery at least half charged.

12. Do not keep mobile phone pressed to ears. Hold it as far as possible and prefer to use a wired earphone or speaker function.

13. Avoid staring for long time into the mobile phone screen, reading large amount of texts, playing games etc as it dries the eyes leading to eye damage.

14. Avoid using mobile phone around other electronics as it increases or focus the radiations.

15. People wearing pacemaker, sunglasses with metal rims, metal wired bras, tooth filling, knee implants etc should minimize, if not possible to avoid completely, the use of mobile phones.

16. Open and empty spaces should be preferred to make longer calls.

17. Avoid owning multiple mobiles or multiple SIM card based mobiles.

18. Avoid using mobile phone inside moving vehicle as the mobile phone signal intensity changes with distance from base tower and metal body of the vehicle traps the signal, which increases the exposure levels.

19. Mobile phone use is banned during driving as it can easily lead to accidents.

20. Children have thinner skulls. Hence children should be completely refrained from mobile phone use. Further, as children are likely to use mobile phones for longer time, lifetime cumulative absorption of radiations will be much higher, which can lead to serious health effects during older age.

21. Mobile phone signals can enter the developing child inside pregnant women; hence mobile phone should be avoided during pregnancy.

22. Use a handbag to carry mobile phone.

ロロロロ

References and Further Reading

CHAPTER 1

1. "Committed to Connecting the World." ITU Releases Latest Global Technology Development Figures. N.p., n.d. Web. 27 Mar. 2014. <http://www.itu.int/net/pressoffice/press_re leases/2012/70.aspx#.UzQQrc5pCHM>.

2. "Jan23 2014Cell Phone Statistics: Updated 2013 Maranda Gibson." *Cell Phone Statistics: Updated 2013*. N.p., n.d. Web. 27 Mar. 2014. <http://www.accuconference.com/blog/Cell-Phone-Statistics.aspx>.

3. "Mind Blowing Cellphone Statistics." The Griffin Technology Blog. N.p., n.d. Web. 25 Mar. 2014. <http://griffintechnology.com/blog/fun/min d-blowing-cellphone-statistics/>.

4. "Mobile Device / Cell Phone Statistics." *Statistic Brain RSS*. N.p., n.d. Web. 27 Mar. 2014.

<http://www.statisticbrain.com/mobile-device-cell-phone-statistics/>.

5. "Mobile Technology Fact Sheet." *Pew Research Centers Internet American Life Project RSS*. N.p., n.d. Web. 24 Mar. 2014. <http://www.pewinternet.org/fact-sheets/mobile-technology-fact-sheet/>.

6. "Nokia 1100." *Wikipedia*. Wikimedia Foundation, 18 Mar. 2014. Web. 27 Mar. 2014. <http://en.wikipedia.org/wiki/Nokia_1100>.

7. "Vision Statement: How People Really Use Mobile." Harvard Business Review. N.p., Jan.-Feb. 2013. Web. 27 Mar. 2014. <http://hbr.org/2013/01/how-people-really-use-mobile/ar/1>.

8. BBC. "Schools Ban Mobile Phones." BBC News. BBC, 01 Aug. 2002. Web. 27 Mar. 2014. <http://news.bbc.co.uk/2/hi/uk_news/education/1748527.stm>.

9. Chowdhury, Rahul. "Evolution of Mobile Phones: 1995 – 2012." *Hongkiatcom RSS*. N.p., n.d. Web. 27 Mar. 2014. <http://www.hongkiat.com/blog/evolution-of-mobile-phones/>.

10. IARC classifies radiofrequency electromagnetic fields as possibly carcinogenic to humans. www.iarc.fr/en/media-centre/pr/2011/pdfs/pr208_E.pdf

11. Kling, Andrew A. Cell Phones. Farmington Hills, MI: Lucent Books, 2010. Print.

12. Phillips, Nicky. "On Mars, the Power of Curiosity Is ... Less than Half a Smartphone." The Sydney Morning Herald. N.p., 09 Aug. 2012. Web. 27 Mar. 2014. <http://www.smh.com.au/technology/sci-tech/on-mars--the-power-of-curiosity-is--less-than-half-a-smartphone-20120809-23wby.html>.

13. Teixeira, Tania. "Meet Marty Cooper - the Inventor of the Mobile Phone." *BBC News*. BBC, 23 Apr. 2010. Web. 27 Mar. 2014. <http://news.bbc.co.uk/2/hi/programmes/click_online/8639590.stm>.

CHAPTER 2

1. Bames, F. S., and B. Greenebaum. "Handbook of Biological Effects of Electromagnetic Fields." (2006).

2. Behari, J. "Biological Responses of Mobile Phone Frequency Exposure." Indian Journal of Experimental Biology. 48.10 (2010): 959-81. Print.

3. Cucurachi, S., et al. "A review of the ecological effects of radiofrequency electromagnetic fields (RF-EMF)." Environment international 51 (2013): 116-140.

4. Current trends in health and safety risk assessment of work related exposure to EMFs. Milan, February 14-16, 2007. Kari Jokela, Non-Ionizing Radiation Laboratory, STUK, Radiation and Nuclear Safety Authority (Finland)

5. Global Mobile Consumer Survey. http://assets.fiercemarkets.net/public/newsletter/fiercewireless/deloitte2013.pdf

6. Grandolfo, M, Sol M. Michaelson, and Alessandro Rindi. Biological Effects and Dosimetry of Nonionizing Radiation: Radiofrequency and Microwave Energies. New York: Published in cooperation with NATO Scientific Affairs Division [by] Plenum Press, 1983. Print.

7. Hantula, Richard. How Do Cell Phones Work?New York, NY: Chelsea Clubhouse, 2009. Print.

8. Higgins, Nadia, and Glen Mullaly. How Cell Phones Work. Mankato, MN: Child's World, 2012. Print.

9. Hosain, Md Kamal. "Effects of Electromagnetic Fields on Mammalian Cells." International Journal of Electrical and Computer Engineering (IJECE) 2.2 (2012): 267-276.

10. Juutilainen, Jukka, et al. "Review of possible modulation-dependent biological effects of radiofrequency fields." Bioelectromagnetics 32.7 (2011): 511-534.

11. Nageswari, K. Sri, and Building Sector. "Biological effects of microwaves and mobile telephony." Proceeding of the

international conference on Non-Ionizing radiation (ICNIR 2003). 2003.

CHAPTER 3

Fitness

1. Carlo, George Louis, and Martin Schram. Cell phones: Invisible hazards in the wireless age. Basic Books, 2002.
2. Davis, Devra. Disconnect: The truth about cell phone radiation, what the industry is doing to hide it, and how to protect your family. Penguin, 2010.
3. Gittleman, PhD, and Ann Louise. "Zapped." New York City: Harper Collins (2010).
4. Ngo, Connie, Richard Porter, and Make an Appointment. "Health Tip 9. Disconnect from EMF. There's a reason to be concerned."
5. Rees, Camilla, and Magda Havas. "Public Health SOS." Wide Angle Health (2008).

Joint problems

1. Berolo, Sophia, Richard P. Wells, and Benjamin C. Amick III. "Musculoskeletal symptoms among mobile hand-held device users and their relationship to device use: A preliminary study in a Canadian university population." Applied Ergonomics 42.2 (2011): 371-378.

2. Darowish, Michael, Jeffrey N. Lawton, and Peter J. Evans. "Q: What is cell phone elbow, and what should we tell our patients?." Cleveland Clinic journal of medicine 76.5 (2009): 306-308.

3. Gustafsson, Ewa, Peter W. Johnson, and Mats Hagberg. "Thumb postures and physical loads during mobile phone use–A comparison of young adults with and without musculoskeletal symptoms." Journal of Electromyography and Kinesiology 20.1 (2010): 127-135.

4. Gustafsson, Ewa. "Ergonomic recommendations when texting on mobile phones." Work: A Journal of Prevention, Assessment and Rehabilitation 41 (2012): 5705-5706.

5. Kennedy, Byron S. "Texting tendinitis in a teenager."

6. Kim, Dong-Soo, and Woen-Sik Chae. "Biomechanical analysis of a smartphone task with different postures." Korean Journal of Sport Biomechanics 22.2 (2012): 253-259.

7. Kim, Gyu Yong, et al. "Effects of the Use of Smartphones on Pain and Muscle Fatigue in the Upper Extremity." Journal of Physical Therapy Science 24.12 (2012): 1255-1258.

8. Ming, Zhiyong, Seppo Pietikainen, and Osmo Hänninen. "Excessive texting in pathophysiology of first carpometacarpal joint arthritis." Pathophysiology 13.4 (2006): 269-270.

9. Nathan-Roberts, Dan, Alex Beeker, and Yili Liu. "Modeling Two Key Physical Ergonomic Problems with Mobile Phones." 2009 University of Michigan Engineering Graduate Symposium. November. 2009.

Hearing loss

1. Christensen, Helle Collatz, et al. "Cellular telephone use and risk of acoustic neuroma." American Journal of Epidemiology 159.3 (2004): 277-283.

2. Hardell, Lennart, et al. "Vestibular schwannoma, tinnitus and cellular telephones." Neuroepidemiology 22.2 (2003): 124-129.

3. Lönn, Stefan, et al. "Mobile phone use and the risk of acoustic neuroma." Epidemiology 15.6 (2004): 653-659.

4. Muscat, J. E., et al. "Handheld cellular telephones and risk of acoustic neuroma." Neurology 58.8 (2002): 1304-1306.

5. Oktay, M. Faruk, and Suleyman Dasdag. "Effects of intensive and moderate cellular phone use on hearing function." Electromagnetic biology and medicine 25.1 (2006): 13-21.

6. Ozturan, Orhan, et al. "Effects of the electromagnetic field of mobile telephones on hearing." Acta oto-laryngologica 122.3 (2002): 289-293.

Ringing ear (Tinnitus)

1. Frei, Patrizia, et al. "Cohort study on the effects of everyday life radio frequency electromagnetic field exposure on non-specific symptoms and tinnitus." Environment international 38.1 (2012): 29-36.

2. Hocking, B. "Preliminary report: symptoms associated with mobile phone use." Occupational Medicine 48.6 (1998): 357-360.

3. Hocking, B. "Preliminary report: symptoms associated with mobile phone use." Occupational Medicine 48.6 (1998): 357-360.

4. Hutter, Hans-Peter, et al. "Tinnitus and mobile phone use." Occupational and environmental medicine 67.12 (2010): 804-808.

Eye damage

1. Balci, Mehmet, Erdinc Devrim, and Ilker Durak. "Effects of mobile phones on oxidant/antioxidant balance in cornea and lens of rats." Current eye research 32.1 (2007): 21-25.

2. Balik, Hasan H., et al. "Some ocular symptoms and sensations experienced by long term users of mobile phones." Pathologie Biologie 53.2 (2005): 88-91.

3. Bormusov, Elvira, et al. "Non-thermal electromagnetic radiation damage to lens epithelium." The open ophthalmology journal 2 (2007): 102-106.

4. Hässig, M., et al. "Prevalence of nuclear cataract in Swiss veal calves and its possible association with mobile telephone antenna base stations." Schweizer Archiv für Tierheilkunde 151.10 (2009): 471-478.

5. Küçer, Nermin. "Some ocular symptoms experienced by users of mobile phones." Electromagnetic biology and medicine 27.2 (2008): 205-209.

6. Lixia, Sun, et al. "Effects of 1.8 GHz radiofrequency field on DNA damage and expression of heat shock protein 70 in human lens epithelial cells." Mutation Research/Fundamental and Molecular Mechanisms of Mutagenesis 602.1 (2006): 135-142.

7. Meo, Sultan A., and Andul M. Al-Dreess. "Mobile phone related hazards and subjective hearing and vision symptoms in

the Saudi population." International journal of occupational medicine and environmental health 18.1 (2005): 45-49.

8. Santini, Roger, et al. "Symptoms experienced by users of digital cellular phones: a study of a french engineering school." Electromagnetic biology and medicine 21.1 (2002): 81-88.

Headache and migraine

1. Al-Khlaiwi, Thamir, and Sultan A. Meo. "Association of mobile phone radiation with fatigue, headache, dizziness, tension and sleep disturbance in Saudi population." Saudi medical journal 25.6 (2004): 732-736.

2. Balikci, Kemal, et al. "A survey study on some neurological symptoms and sensations experienced by long term users of mobile phones." Pathologie Biologie 53.1 (2005): 30-34.

3. Hocking, B. "Preliminary report: symptoms associated with mobile phone use." Occupational Medicine 48.6 (1998): 357-360.

4. Oftedal, Gunnhild, et al. "Mobile phone headache: a double blind, sham-controlled

provocation study." Cephalalgia 27.5 (2007): 447-455.

5. Schüz, Joachim, et al. "Risks for central nervous system diseases among mobile phone subscribers: a Danish retrospective cohort study." PLoS One 4.2 (2009): e4389.

Pedestrian injury

1. Hatfield, Julie, and Susanne Murphy. "The effects of mobile phone use on pedestrian crossing behaviour at signalised and unsignalised intersections." Accident Analysis & Prevention 39.1 (2007): 197-205.

2. Nasar, Jack, Peter Hecht, and Richard Wener. "Mobile telephones, distracted attention, and pedestrian safety." Accident Analysis & Prevention 40.1 (2008): 69-75.

3. Stavrinos, Despina, Katherine W. Byington, and David C. Schwebel. "Effect of cell phone distraction on pediatric pedestrian injury risk." Pediatrics 123.2 (2009): e179-e185.

Fatigue

1. Al-Khlaiwi, Thamir, and Sultan A. Meo. "Association of mobile phone radiation with fatigue, headache, dizziness, tension and sleep disturbance in Saudi population." Saudi medical journal 25.6 (2004): 732-736.

2. Sandström, M., et al. "Mobile phone use and subjective symptoms. Comparison of symptoms experienced by users of analogue and digital mobile phones." Occupational Medicine 51.1 (2001): 25-35.

3. Thomée, Sara, Annika Härenstam, and Mats Hagberg. "Mobile phone use and stress, sleep disturbances, and symptoms of depression among young adults-a prospective cohort study." BMC public health 11.1 (2011): 66.

4. Thomée, Sara, et al. "Prevalence of perceived stress, symptoms of depression and sleep disturbances in relation to information and communication technology (ICT) use among young adults–an explorative prospective study." Computers in Human Behavior 23.3 (2007): 1300-1321.

Skin allergy

1. Kimata, H. "Enhancement of allergic skin wheal responses in patients with atopic eczema/dermatitis syndrome by playing video games or by a frequently ringing mobile phone." European journal of clinical investigation 33.6 (2003): 513-517.

2. Kimata, Hajime. "Enhancement of allergic skin wheal responses by microwave radiation from mobile phones in patients with atopic eczema/dermatitis syndrome." International archives of allergy and immunology 129.4 (2002): 348-350.

3. Roberts, Hugh, and Bruce Tate. "Nickel allergy presenting as mobile phone contact dermatitis." Australasian Journal of Dermatology 51.1 (2010): 23-25.

4. Seishima, Mariko, Zuiei Oyama, and Makiko Oda. "Cellular phone dermatitis with chromate allergy." Dermatology 207.1 (2003): 48-50.

5. Wohrl, Stefan, et al. "Mobile telephone as new source for nickel dermatitis." Contact Dermatitis 56.2 (2007): 113.

Weakening of the Blood brain barrier & changes in the brain activity

1. Croft, Rodney J., et al. "Acute mobile phone operation affects neural function in humans." Clinical Neurophysiology 113.10 (2002): 1623-1632.

2. Eberhardt, Jacob L., et al. "Blood-brain barrier permeability and nerve cell damage in rat brain 14 and 28 days after exposure to microwaves from GSM mobile phones." Electromagnetic biology and medicine 27.3 (2008): 215-229.

3. Eulitz, Carsten, et al. "Mobile phones modulate response patterns of human brain activity." Neuroreport 9.14 (1998): 3229-3232.

4. Hamblin, D. L., and A. W. Wood. "Effects of mobile phone emissions on human brain activity and sleep variables." International journal of radiation biology 78.8 (2002): 659-669.

5. Leszczynski, Dariusz, et al. "Non-thermal activation of the hsp27/p38MAPK stress pathway by mobile phone radiation in human endothelial cells: molecular mechanism for cancer-and blood-brain

barrier-related effects." Differentiation 70.2 (2002): 120-129.

6. Leszczynski, Dariusz. "Mobile Phones and Blood-Brain Barrier."

7. Nittby, Henrietta, et al. "Increased blood–brain barrier permeability in mammalian brain 7 days after exposure to the radiation from a GSM-900 mobile phone." Pathophysiology 16.2 (2009): 103-112.

8. Salford, Leif G., et al. "Nerve cell damage in mammalian brain after exposure to microwaves from GSM mobile phones." Environmental health perspectives 111.7 (2003): 881.

9. Volkow, Nora D., et al. "Effects of cell phone radiofrequency signal exposure on brain glucose metabolism." Jama 305.8 (2011): 808-813.

Erectile dysfunction

1. Proceedings of the World Meeting on Sexual Medicine. (August 2, 2012). The Journal of Sexual Medicine. doi: 10.1111/j.1743-6109.2012.02863.x

2. "Physicians Believe Smartphones Can Trigger Impotence." Erectile Doctor. N.p., n.d. Web. 27 Mar. 2014.

Male infertility

1. Agarwal, Ashok, et al. "Effect of cell phone usage on semen analysis in men attending infertility clinic: an observational study." Fertility and sterility 89.1 (2008): 124-128.

2. Aitken, R. J., et al. "Impact of radio frequency electromagnetic radiation on DNA integrity in the male germline." International journal of andrology 28.3 (2005): 171-179.

3. Dama, Madhukar Shivajirao, and M. Narayana Bhat. "Mobile phones affect multiple sperm quality traits." (2013).

4. De Iuliis, Geoffry N., et al. "Mobile phone radiation induces reactive oxygen species production and DNA damage in human spermatozoa in vitro." PLoS One 4.7 (2009): e6446.

5. Deepinder, Fnu, Kartikeya Makker, and Ashok Agarwal. "Cell phones and male infertility: dissecting the relationship."

Reproductive biomedicine online 15.3
(2007): 266-270.

6. Wdowiak, Artur, Leszek Wdowiak, and
Henryk Wiktor. "Evaluation of the effect of
using mobile phones on male fertility."
Annals of Agricultural and Environmental
Medicine 14.1 (2007): 169-172.

Sleep disturbance, confusion, mood swings, stress & depression

1. Al-Khlaiwi, Thamir, and Sultan A. Meo.
"Association of mobile phone radiation with
fatigue, headache, dizziness, tension and
sleep disturbance in Saudi population."
Saudi medical journal 25.6 (2004): 732-736.

2. Progress in Electromagnetics Research
Symposium 2008: (piers 2008 Hangzhou);
Hangzhou, China, 24 - 28 March 2008. Red
Hook, NY: Curran, 2011. Print.

3. Progress in Electromagnetics Research
Symposium 2008: (piers 2008 Cambridge) ;
Cambridge, Massachusetts, Usa, 2 - 6 July
2008. Red Hook, NY: Curran, 2011. Print.

4. Thomée, Sara, Annika Härenstam, and Mats
Hagberg. "Mobile phone use and stress,

sleep disturbances, and symptoms of depression among young adults-a prospective cohort study." BMC public health 11.1 (2011): 66.

Annoyance

1. End, Christian M., et al. "Costly cell phones: The impact of cell phone rings on academic performance." Teaching of Psychology 37.1 (2009): 55-57.
2. Monk, Andrew, et al. "Why are mobile phones annoying?." Behaviour & Information Technology 23.1 (2004): 33-41.
3. Monk, Andrew, Evi Fellas, and Eleanor Ley. "Hearing only one side of normal and mobile phone conversations." Behaviour & Information Technology 23.5 (2004): 301-305.
4. Shelton, Jill T., et al. "The distracting effects of a ringing cell phone: An investigation of the laboratory and the classroom setting." Journal of Environmental Psychology 29.4 (2009): 513-521.
5. Turner, Mark, Steve Love, and Mark Howell. "Understanding emotions

experienced when using a mobile phone in public: The social usability of mobile (cellular) telephones." Telematics and Informatics 25.3 (2008): 201-215.

Distracted driving and traffic accidents

1. Alm, Håkan, and Lena Nilsson. "The effects of a mobile telephone task on driver behaviour in a car following situation." Accident Analysis & Prevention 27.5 (1995): 707-715.

2. Brookhuis, Karel A., Gerbrand de Vries, and Dick de Waard. "The effects of mobile telephoning on driving performance." Accident Analysis & Prevention 23.4 (1991): 309-316.

3. Hancock, P. A., M. Lesch, and Lisa Simmons. "The distraction effects of phone use during a crucial driving maneuver." Accident Analysis & Prevention 35.4 (2003): 501-514.

4. Horberry, Tim, et al. "Driver distraction: the effects of concurrent in-vehicle tasks, road

environment complexity and age on driving performance." Accident Analysis & Prevention 38.1 (2006): 185-191.

5. http://en.wikipedia.org/wiki/Mobile_phones_and_driving_safety

6. http://www.edgarsnyder.com/

7. McKnight, A. James, and A. Scott McKnight. "The effect of cellular phone use upon driver attention." Accident Analysis & Prevention 25.3 (1993): 259-265.

Killing communication skills

1. "4 Ways Texting Is Killing Our Communication Skills." Main. N.p., n.d. Web. 27 Mar. 2014.

2. "Does Cell Phone Use Really Affect Our Communication Skills?" The Lance. N.p., n.d. Web. 26 Mar. 2014.

3. "Lost in Translation: Texting Killing Human Communication Skills." The DePaulia. N.p., n.d. Web. 27 Mar. 2014.

<http://www.depauliaonline.com/opinions/l
ost-in-translation-texting-killing-human-
communication-skills-1.2841429#.UzPL-
c5pCHM>.

4. Campbell, Scott W., and Nojin Kwak.
    "Mobile communication and civil society:
    Linking patterns and places of use to
    engagement with others in public." Human
    Communication Research 37.2 (2011): 207-
    222.

5. Ling, Rich, and Scott W. Campbell, eds.
    Mobile communication: Bringing us
    together and tearing us apart. Vol. 1.
    Transaction Publishers, 2011.

Affecting socialization

1. Campbell, Scott W., and Nojin Kwak.
    "Mobile communication and civil society:
    Linking patterns and places of use to
    engagement with others in public." Human
    Communication Research 37.2 (2011): 207-
    222.

2. Ling, Rich, and Scott W. Campbell, eds.

Mobile communication: Bringing us together and tearing us apart. Vol. 1. Transaction Publishers, 2011.

Predisposition to Selfishness & Criminality

1. "University of Winnipeg | News Centre." UWinnipeg News Centre Study Supports Theory On Teen Texting And Shallow Thought Comments. N.p., n.d. Web. 27 Mar. 2014. <http://news-centre.uwinnipeg.ca/all-posts/study-supports-theory-on-teen-texting-and-shallow-thought/>.

2. Abraham, Ajay T., Anastasiya Pocheptsova, and Rosellina Ferraro. "The effect of mobile phone use on prosocial behavior." Unpublished manuscript, University of Maryland (2012).

3. Sherman, Megan. "Sixteen, sexting, and a sex offender: how advances in cell phone technology have led to teenage sex offenders." BUJ Sci. & Tech. L. 17 (2011): 138.

Behavioural problems

1. "One-fifth of Third-graders Own Cell Phones." CNET. N.p., n.d. Web. 24 Mar. 2014. <http://www.cnet.com/news/one-fifth-of-third-graders-own-cell-phones/>.

2. Divan, Hozefa A., et al. "Cell phone use and behavioural problems in young children." Journal of epidemiology and community health 66.6 (2012): 524-529.

3. Divan, Hozefa A., et al. "Prenatal and postnatal exposure to cell phone use and behavioral problems in children." Epidemiology 19.6 (2008): S94-S95.

4. Divan, Hozefa A., Leeka Kheifets, and Jørn Olsen. "Prenatal cell phone use and developmental milestone delays among infants." Scandinavian journal of work, environment & health (2011): 341-348.

5. Guxens, Mònica, et al. "Maternal cell phone and cordless phone use during pregnancy and behaviour problems in 5-year-old children." Journal of epidemiology and community health 67.5 (2013): 432-438.

6. http://www.pewinternet.org/Reports/2013/Teens-and-Tech.aspx

7. Vrijheid, Martine, et al. "Prenatal exposure to cell phone use and neurodevelopment at 14 months." Epidemiology 21.2 (2010): 259-262.

Cancers

1. IARC classifies radiofrequency electromagnetic fields as possibly carcinogenic to humans. www.iarc.fr/en/media-centre/pr/2011/pdfs/pr208_E.pdf

2. Johansen, Christoffer, et al. "Cellular telephones and cancer—a nationwide cohort study in Denmark." Journal of the National Cancer Institute 93.3 (2001): 203-207.

¤¤¤¤¤

Acknowledgements

Research on the harmful effects of cell phone are either ignored or ridiculed. Despite this, hundreds of scientists are working undeterred. I salute them.

First and foremost, I thank Prof. H. A. Upendra, whose guidance and support was instrumental in initiating this project. Though, neither I can explain *how it happened*, nor he could *realize his role*.

Then, during all the stages of writing, many discussions happened with friends, which shaped my ideas. Most important was Sangshetty Balkunde Ramona Coates, and Dr. Ayyappa, who corrected my drafts honestly. It was friends at Rotary Kushalnagar, especially, Dr. Dharanendra, Dr. Hari Shetty, Naveen, Shaji KG, Chengappa AA, and all Rotarians, who endorsed my ideas and complemented my thoughts.

I am also very thankful to CreateSpace self publishing platform, which was a crucial factor making me write a book. I am scared of agents and middlemen!

Finally, to Savitri and Adhya, who are my everything.

¤¤¤¤¤

MADHUKAR DAMA

About the Author

Dr. Madhukar Dama is an Assistant Professor and a social worker. After a career in drug discovery, Dr. Madhukar is now dedicated to research, and takes pride in spreading awareness about the hidden dangers of things that we use daily but take for granted. Most importantly, the effects of human activities on our environment and wildlife, and hazards of indiscriminate use of pesticides and misuse of plastics. Microwave contamination of the atmosphere and hazards to a mobile phone user are his current interests.